For my grandparents, Connie and John, who have supported me in more ways than one. For my grandpa, Peter, who passed away during my recovery and for Mike's late father, Martin. Thank you to everyone who has supported me in this journey of recovery. I will be forever grateful to you all.

All proceeds from the sale of this book are donated to SEED - Eating Disorders Support Services (Registered Charity Number: 1108405). For more information and support please visit:

https://seedeatingdisorders.org.uk

First published in 2021 through the

Independent Publishing Network (IPN)

ISBN 978-1-80049-388-9

ED Versus Me

A Journey of Recovery
From An Eating Disorder

by Georgie M. Beadman,
Sally R. Wilkes & Eleanor F. Brogan

Introduction

This book was written twenty-eight months after Georgie first admitted that she needed help. Unbeknown to all, she had been suffering with an eating disorder for many, many years. You may wonder how it is that no one knew. Well Georgie was a master of disguise. A vibrant, enthusiastic and outgoing person, you would never have suspected that she was going through so much turmoil inside. Had she not finally admitted it, we would probably have gone on not suspecting a thing until it was too late.

The aim of the book is to provide an honest account of what it's like to live with an eating disorder both from Georgie's perspective and that of her two friends Eleanor (Ellie) and Sally. Ellie first met Georgie at university and has known her for over seven years now.

Sally met Mike, Georgie's partner on her first day at university. He lived in the flat below her and over the next three years they became good friends. It just so happened that he was also good friends with her now husband and was the best man at their wedding. Mike met Georgie just over a year before Georgie's diagnosis and not long before Sally gave birth to her first child, something which Sally and Georgie bonded over in the coming years.

To set the scene a little more, Georgie was first diagnosed with an eating disorder by a General Practitioner (GP) in January 2018 at the age of twenty-five. She was put on a waiting list for an NHS eating disorder clinic but was told that she would have to wait until the end of May 2018 for an appointment. By this point Georgie was seriously ill and we can't even begin to think about what the outcome would have been if she had waited that long. Georgie was extremely fortunate in that she was able to access private care which shortened this wait significantly. That is not to say that her journey from there on was easy. Far from it.

For the next seven months Georgie could not be left on her own. This meant that it was not only a challenging time for Georgie but also for those around her. She was put on a strict diet and all exercise was forbidden and so someone needed to be with her at all times to enforce this. To help drown out the voice of the eating disorder which was telling her to do the opposite.

Georgie voiced several times during this period that she felt like a burden but none of us saw her as that in the slightest. Georgie was, and still is, the happiest, kindest, most loving person we all know. She would do anything for anyone and so to us, helping her to recover from this life-threatening illness was the very least we could do. And that's exactly what it is. Just like cancer, an eating disorder attacks your mind, body and soul and if left untreated it will eventually kill you. We refer to Georgie's eating disorder throughout the book as 'ED' as this is the name Georgie has since given to the monster that resided in her head for so long.

There were two weeks early on where Georgie's family couldn't physically be at her side and Georgie's partner, Mike, couldn't take any more time off work. And so, Ellie moved in with Georgie during that time. However, not once did Ellie see herself as a carer during those two weeks. From March 2018, Georgie also started spending a day or two each week at Sally's house with her 18-month-old daughter. Sally found her presence a huge help as she was and still is brilliant with children and, as someone who was desperate for children of her own, this was the ultimate motivation for Georgie to get better.

And she did just that! In the battle of ED versus Georgie, she has won and she is now weeks away from being fully discharged. Georgie couldn't work for a long time but she now has her dream job working in a school for disadvantaged children, once again showing just how kind and caring she is. Her and Mike also have plans for a big adventure travelling the world this summer. It has been a long road to recovery but she is now living her life to the full. And so, in the words of Georgie's favourite quote...no rain, no flowers!

If you are reading this book then you too are most probably living with or have lived with an eating disorder. We didn't want to write something that was draining to read, especially given you probably already feel drained both physically and emotionally. For that reason, we have written it in such a way that should make it easy to dip in and out. The book is split into two sections - one written from Georgie's perspective and the other from that of Ellie and Sally. Each section is further broken down into smaller sections consisting of a short poem followed by two pages of text that go into more detail.

We realise that our experiences of living with an eating disorder will not be the same as everyone else's. We also fully acknowledge that not everyone is able to access private care. Georgie, her family and her friends will all be forever thankful that she was in a position to access such care. We are now determined to do everything in our power to change things for the better and so all proceeds from this book will go towards supporting others suffering with an eating disorder.

I Can

I Will

I Did

Run Eat
Run Repeat

The light is shining through my curtains,
I must get up and run.
I have no time for breakfast,
A sip of water and I'm done.

At least an hour's worth of running,
Before my work day can begin.
I'll be forced to work with Anna.
God I wish I was that thin.

Two rice cakes now for lunch.
Perhaps a treat of something fruity.
There's not much time to sit though,
It's my turn for playground duty.

Tonight we'll eat fish fingers,
But first another run.
If I run a little bit further,
I'll be allowed more than just one.

Tomorrow is the weekend.
It means I have more time for me.
I can run for several hours,
My reward will be TV.

I wish I had more time for running,
To be the best version of me.
Instead, I look in the mirror,
And I hate all that I see.

This was my life. It makes me so sad when I look back on how my days used to be ruled by my next 'hit' of exercise.

My favourite time of day used to be going to bed for the simple reason that I could rest my body and mind without the 'lazy, fat, ugly, worthless' thoughts running constantly through my head. I used to spend hours awake on my phone looking at hints and tips for how to lose weight and how to be as fit as possible. That sentence is wrong in so many different ways. How can you be as fit as possible whilst losing as much weight as possible? That's like trying to run a marathon as fast as you can but with no fuel. It just won't work.

My partner, Mike, found it extremely hard at weekends as I would be in a really foul mood unless I had been running for at least two hours. We had many, many arguments over this and looking back it scares me thinking about how easily I was able to justify all of it to myself. I genuinely convinced myself that it was normal. I now understand that it was all part of my eating disorder. ED's voice in my head was so strong. He was doing his best to alienate me from everyone that cared. To make me feel angry towards those who loved me and jealous of all my friends. I stopped wanting to socialise and hated going out for meals. I had no confidence and felt as though no one could really want me around.

I'm a qualified primary school teacher, something that I am extremely proud of. All throughout my childhood, I struggled at school with dyslexia and dyspraxia and so I never even contemplated that I could make it as a teacher. But here I am, proof that you should never let anyone or anything stop you reaching your dreams. I had the job of my dreams in a small village primary school as the nursery/reception class teacher. I loved the children and my team and every day was an adventure.

Having said all this, I found work very hard and continually struggled. This was not with the workload, the staff or the children as most people might expect. It was the thought of doing activities at the table with the children. I hated sitting down. This next bit is something I hate to admit as I love reading and think that it's such an important skill. I am ashamed to say that even when children were reading to me all I could hear was the voice in my head telling me I was lazy for sitting down and my punishment would be no lunch. It's crazy when I think back as I can now see how unhealthy and damaging those thoughts were.

Underneath it all, I just wanted to feel 'normal' whatever normal might be. The truth was I hated my repetitive life and I just wanted to scream 'STOP!'

But I'm

Intolerant

I'm not getting any thinner,
I still look fricking fat.
Could it be what I am eating?
Yes I think it must be that.

I'm intolerant to lactose,
So it's not like I eat cheese.
And gluten gives me tummy ache,
So I'll cut out carbs with ease.

I've been checking out the calories,
In things I normally eat.
Fish fingers are a high one,
Along with any type of meat.

I've cut out all the sugars,
Even fruit is bad for me.
Diet Coke now keeps me going,
At least that's sugar free.

Vegetables and vitamin pills,
That's what I eat now.
But I still have loads of fat to lose,
And I really don't know how.

Tomorrow I'll do better,
I'll try eat even less.
I'll take comfort from my hunger.
It's a step towards success.

I remember when I first started getting tummy aches every time I ate. I was about fifteen or sixteen years old and my tummy used to bloat up to three times the size. I used to call it my 'food baby'. My parents took me to see a specialist and they put me on several different diets. The one that worked for me was no lactose (basically anything tasty) and no gluten (basically anything tasty). I say this meaning no disrespect to those who genuinely can't eat such items, as I know there are now plenty of great alternatives out there.

I avoided eating all gluten and then I cut dairy out too. I literally just ate protein and vegetables - how boring is that!? I went all the way through university without having a McDonald's or cheesy chips after a night out. I don't care how 'healthy' you claim to be, everybody loves cheesy chips after dancing all night. This is just one example of an experience that ED robbed from me.

I went to countless restaurants and missed out on endless delicious meals choosing to order a salad (with no dressing, cheese or croutons). Salads are great but not when it is quite literally limp lettuce and dry chicken. I missed out on the full experience of a girl's night as I avoided all chocolate, crisps and pizza. My family and I went on a cycling holiday around Italy and whilst everyone else was fueled with fresh Italian pasta and pizza I was fueled with free peanuts (you know, the tiny cup full you get in some countries when you order a drink) and boring salads. I can assure you I would have experienced far more on this holiday if I had eaten the local cuisine. It makes me sad to look back on all the experiences that I missed all because ED somehow convinced me that I was fat and worthless.

It gets worse! Fast forward a few years and ED then decided that meat was also "bad". I put the word bad in inverted commas because I now strongly believe that there is no good or bad when it comes to food and I refuse to even say it when talking about the past. I basically lived on a diet that consisted only of vegetables and sugar free vitamin pills. I won't go into any more details than I already have as I don't want anyone reading this to think that it sounds like a good diet to try. It 100% is not!!

If you get squeamish I suggest you skip ahead the next few lines. Don't ever try this diet!! In fact, don't try any diet for that matter. The diet industry is worth over £2 billion in the UK alone. It's no wonder that they tell everyone what the "perfect" body should look like and how you can try to get it! Anyway, rant over! This disgusting diet gives you the worst stomach pains ever. My stomach swelled to its maximum on a daily basis. I genuinely could have passed for being forty weeks pregnant! You then have the worst time sitting in excruciating pain on the toilet for at least half an hour before standing up only to have to go again. I was disgusted by myself and felt so ashamed. I remember my stomach once swelled so much that it hurt to breathe. This was when I realised how serious things had become.

Master Of

Disguises

It feels like all the friends I have,
Are different to me.
But I cannot let them know this,
I cannot let them see.

I hate just sitting still,
I'm always busy, this is true.
But I don't like what they're watching,
And I've things I need to do.

Some ask why I eat starters,
Instead of ordering mains.
But I can't eat those ingredients,
They give me stomach pains.

Leggings and baggy jumpers,
My go to style since my late teens.
But I don't suit what they're all wearing,
Tiny tops and skinny jeans.

I'm tired of people asking,
"Why'd you run so much?" they say.
Now I stop and run on my drive home,
"There was traffic on the way."

I worry if I break my cover,
I'll be a freak in all their eyes.
So, I'll continue as I have been.
I'll become a master of disguise.

University was a hard time for me in many ways. I quit the first time around as I was miserable - it was definitely ED. Then I started again in York a few years later to do my Primary Education degree. I wasn't aware that I was poorly at the time but ED's voice was definitely there. However, as anyone who knew me then will tell you, I was the master of disguise. I did everything I possibly could to hide any sign of ED.

Looking back, there were quite a few red flags. I would always order a starter portion of food. I would never want to sit down and eat lunch. I had to go for a run every day, even before a 9am lecture - what student does that! And you would never see me wearing jeans, always leggings and loose ones at that.

Let me tell you a little bit more about 'the jean phobia'. It sounds ridiculous, I know, but I think the reasons behind it were key to my illness. I used to look at everyone in the street wearing jeans and wish I could be just like them. But ED convinced me that I looked disgusting in them. I spent my teenage years in leggings and this continued into my twenties. The weird thing was that I loved nothing more than the feeling of my leggings hanging off me. Any normal person would throw leggings in the bin when they lost their elasticity but this was when I loved them most.

I remember talking about this with my psychologist and in the end, we linked it with a memory from when I was 15 and going away with my school. About two months before I was due to go away, I had bought some non-stretchy trousers to wear. When the day came, I found that my trousers didn't fit. You can imagine how that made me feel. I had to wear a belt to stop then from falling down as I couldn't even do up the button. It was humiliating, especially when I so desperately wanted to fit in with my peers. This experience affected me more than I first realised as it was on this trip that I first began to get my 'funny tummy'.

I met Mike in my final year of university, on Tinder of all places! I used to enjoy talking to him and for the first time I felt confident, mainly because I was behind a screen and so I didn't feel judged on my appearance. Once we got to know each other more, Mike began to question me about my eating and exercise habits. I would always just sweep it under the carpet with ' I just love to run, there is nothing wrong with that'. Mike was wearing rose tinted glasses at this point so would go along with what I said.

These conversations got more intense when we moved in together. I would consistently miss breakfast, try to escape lunch and then be late for dinner most weeknights as I was too busy running. I still managed to convince him that all this was okay. That I just didn't like eating in a morning. That I'd had a meeting after work, not that I'd actually run seven miles on the way home. It wasn't until I admitted I needed help that the disguise finally fell away. It genuinely felt like a cloak had been lifted and I could finally start to be free.

This Is

No Life

I've just eaten a strawberry.
Why do I feel so bad?
Now I'll have to go and exercise,
To burn what it will add.

I drink water from the vegetables,
To get the nutrients I lack.
I treat vitamin pills like sweeties,
Every day I take a pack.

I've become a master of excuses,
To divert or to defend.
All I really eat are vegetables,
And I run for hours on end.

How can all this be normal?
How can I be alright?
It feels like every single day,
All I do is fight.

I wish I wasn't so fixated,
On trying to be thin.
I want to enjoy my life,
And feel happier within.

I'm not sure I have the energy,
To carry on this way.
Maybe I should tell someone,
But then, what would I say?

The day I want to call 'strawberry day' started off as usual - a long run, no breakfast and no liquids. I then headed straight out for a long walk at one of my favourite places in the world, Bradgate Park. If you have never been here then I recommend adding it to your bucket list! It's a beautiful, old deer park that has barely been touched since Lady Jane Grey lived there many, many years ago. For any history lovers, she was the shortest reigning queen in England.

Anyway, back to my boring story of the dreaded strawberry... My mum had brought some strawberries along on this beautiful family walk. When I was offered one, I clearly remember thinking I had to take one to avoid any awkward "why aren't you hungry, it's only a strawberry" type questions. I ate one really, really slowly to avoid being offered another one. With each mouthful the voice in my head became stronger. I began to feel heavier and more worthless with every miniscule bite I took.

When I think about this day I want to go back and give myself a good talking to. "It's only a strawberry! Just eat it! You've been for a run and a walk and your body is craving energy". However, the phrase 'just eat it' is enough to send anyone who has suffered or is suffering with an eating disorder into a rage. If it was as easy at that we would be eating!! I knew right then that I needed to do something about this. I was sat in a beautiful park on a sunny day with my very happy and healthy family. I had a secure job and my dream home yet all I could do was worry about the half a strawberry I'd just eaten. This was not okay, and something had to be done.

At the time, if I ever I began to think like this it made ED very angry. His voice would persistently tell me how fat and useless I was. I did my best to ignore it but the voice grew louder and louder with every step taken and with every bite not eaten. With this the need to control my weight also became stronger and stronger.

I Need

Help

I know that I'm hurting myself,
With every step I take.
But the stupid voice that's in my head,
Will not give me a break!

I'm scared of what they'll think of me,
That the voice's words are true.
"People will either take control,
Or worse they'll laugh at you."

But I know I can't go on like this,
Despite the monster in my head.
It's trying to convince me I am normal,
If I listen, I'll soon be dead.

There's a simple word I need to use,
Yet, it's the hardest one to say.
It'll take all the strength I have left,
To say this word today.

My hands are visibly shaking.
My throat is as dry as a bone.
But here I go, "I need your HELP,
I can't do this alone."

I have a new strength inside me,
Where before I felt I had none.
The weight on my shoulders has lifted.
The burden I carried has gone.

It's not easy to think back to the day that I finally asked for help as I can only imagine how it made my partner, Mike, feel. He had just lost his dad after years of traumatic alcohol abuse and here I was, another 'addict' about to take him through round two. It was a Sunday morning, the 5th January to be precise. It was the day after Mike had lost his dad and I woke up at 5am only able to think about whether I could go for a run. Would Mike be mad if I didn't stay in bed to comfort him?

After half an hour of deliberation I got up and began to brush my teeth. I was halfway through my bottom jaw when my mind finally overcame ED's controlling voice. "What am I doing!? Mike has just lost his dad and here I am sneaking off to go for a 12-mile run instead of staying home and looking after him."

I remember getting back into bed and lying awake for hours just thinking about what on Earth was going on in my head. The one thing that kept replaying in my mind was the fact that Mike's dad had finally succumbed to his mental illness and I did not want to do the same. The pain of seeing Mike have to visit his dying father in hospital was unthinkable and I couldn't risk putting him through anything like that again. I had to beat it. For Mike. For his dad.

I never met Mike's dad in person but I'll be forever grateful to him for making me realise that I needed to get my life back on track. Obviously, the day after Mike had lost his dad was not the best timing for me to open up about everything but I didn't want ED to convince me otherwise. I knew it had to be done.

We headed out for a walk and I played over and over in my head what I should say but I couldn't quite open my mouth and say it. This is when the weirdest thing happened. Mike randomly asked, "why do you look so unwell in the picture that your mum and dad have in their kitchen?" Safe to say I just burst into tears.

Telling Mike about ED was really hard. I was scared that he would think I was mad or that he would compare me to his dad and want to run away. But he didn't. He just stayed quiet and listened and by the time we had walked home we had come up with a plan.

I called my parents and he helped me to tell them. I don't think they were surprised as my eating habits had been strange for years. My mum then said that she would drive up the very next day to come with me to see the doctor and to tell my brother, Tom. This was also severely bad timing, as he was weeks away from his finals in his medical degree. Tom actually took it well. We played it down to a certain extent, as we didn't want to worry him. My brother failing his finals was the last thing I needed to have on my conscience. Then it was time to put on my big girl pants and visit the doctor.

A Trip To

The Doctor

The first doctor I saw was just rubbish.
He made me feel silly and vain.
But I've built up my strength and my courage,
To go back to the doctor again.

They've said it's an eating disorder.
From now on I'll call it ED.
I've been put on a list for some clinic,
And they've said they'll monitor me.

I feel better knowing it's been acknowledged.
That I'll be getting the help that I need.
For years this monster's been growing,
Like an out of control garden weed.

I still feel a little bit nervous.
I hope there's not long to wait.
It took all that I had to come forward.
To admit that I'm not doing great.

For now, I'm not sure what the plan is.
I guess it's just wait and see.
All I know is I want my life back.
A life not involving ED.

Walking into the doctor's surgery the day after admitting to my family and Mike that I thought I had a problem felt like the most humiliating day of my life. It was the "can I ask what you wish to see a doctor about?" from the receptionist that filled me with anxiety. The first doctor I saw was rubbish. I hate to call any medical professional rubbish but he was extremely un-sympathetic and in all honesty he made me feel worse. I imagine it was far from what he intended but his lack of concern was abundantly clear. Safe to say I went home and cried.

Thank goodness for Mike and my family. With their help I managed to pluck up the courage to go back to the doctor's and this time I asked for a mental health specialist when they asked the dreaded "why are you here?" question. My mum came with me too. Strangely, I craved to be like a child again, especially in the company of loved ones. It was like I had started to regress in more ways than one. I needed my mum with me to do all the normal adult activities. Any self-confidence I'd gained in my early twenties was long gone.

Anyway, I couldn't have been given a nicer doctor this time. She listened to my concerns, was patient whilst I cried and really took note of what I was saying. This is when I finally got referred to the eating disorders clinic. When I say 'got referred', this actually meant that my name was put on the longest waiting list in the whole entire world. During the next month ED grew so much stronger. It was as though he was thriving from me being on that waiting list. He would tell me that I obviously wasn't poorly as no one thought I needed help urgently. He told me I was still fat and the worst one of all, he used to try and convince me that I had made it all up and that I didn't need any help. If it hadn't been for Mike and my family, it would have been all too easy to cancel my appointment and bow down to ED.

After a month of waiting I had lost enough weight for things to be considered serious. To this day, this still infuriates me. The fact that I was first told I would be put on a waiting list because my BMI was 'okay' just made ED a million times worse. In my head this was the same as the doctor telling me I was fat. This is what made me spiral down, almost like a subconscious cry for help. ED was fueled by the fact that he had 3 months to consume me.

I just want to take a minute to mention my amazing grandparents at this point. They are my heroes in more ways than one. They stepped in when I was most in need and for that, I will be eternally grateful to them both. They helped secure me an appointment, a two-hour drive from where I lived but with only a week's wait. The buildup was hideous. ED pushed me to do as many steps as possible on as little food as possible before any professional could intervene. It was as though I had created a personalised concentration camp for myself. There is no other word I can use to describe that time other than hell.

The

Clinic

My shoes feel full of concrete.
I can't walk through the door.
My head and my mouth are in battle,
With ED saying "speak no more".

No one really gets it.
I'm angry at those I see.
I'm a fraud. I'm not anorexic!
They're wasting their time on me.

The dietician now wants to weigh me.
She thinks I'm being silly no doubt.
She lays me down to take my blood pressure,
As she's worried that I'll pass out.

The news she just told me was brutal.
Your bones are weak, you're wasting away.
Your heart will soon give up on you,
If you carry on this way.

She has said that she can help me,
But ED is not a fan.
He hates her with a passion,
For spoiling his wicked plan.

She wants control of my food and my exercise.
Yet, in some ways I now feel free.
It's going to be quite a challenge,
But right here is the start of ME.

The day I first visited the clinic to see my dietitian was the 23rd February 2018 around eight or nine years after all my strange eating habits had begun. I knew then that this was the start of a long journey to finding me again. I was absolutely terrified. I don't think I said a word throughout the whole car journey. Those who know me will know what a rarity that is! I sat in sweaty silence having a battle in my head with ED.

I just wanted to cancel the appointment or hoped that we wouldn't find the right door. Mike came with me for support. I definitely would have run away or conveniently 'got lost' without him there. We sat and waited for what seemed like forever. When I was finally taken into a room, I wanted Mike to come in too. He was like my comfort blanket and I knew he would help me tell her the truth.

My dietitian was so upbeat and had a great personality that matched perfectly to mine so I immediately felt more at ease. She needed to take my blood pressure and I remember her looking at me and asking me to lie down as she was afraid I would pass out. That's when it really, really hit home. This was scary! A professional was worried that my body wouldn't be able to withstand my blood pressure being taken whilst standing up.

She then told me the terrifying truth. To this day I still find it difficult to comprehend. Even whilst she was telling me the truth, ED's voice was still trying to convince me that there was nothing wrong with me. The words she said were something along the lines of, "This is really serious

Georgie. We need to get some nutrients back into your body as safely as we can. If we do this too quickly your heart won't cope. Your bones are brittle and are wasting away and your body has started to shut down". Thinking back, those words make me shudder.

From that moment onwards my dietitian controlled all that I ate. It was horrible, especially at the start. I was on tiny portions of food, which made my tummy growl with hunger and ED scream with anger. This was to prevent me from going into refeeding syndrome, where my heart would basically shut down unable to cope with eating. I was watched 24/7 and had no privacy whatsoever. Mike even sat and watched me poo - that was the 'honeymoon' stage firmly over! I was angry at food and at the person who gave it to me. This was ED showing his true colours and trying to rule over me once more. But I pushed his voice aside and ate what I was given, killing ED with every miniscule mouthful.

I will be forever thankful to my mum who made the seemingly endless trips with me to and from the clinic every week. And also for the never-ending and much needed love and support from the rest of my family, Mike, his mum, his step dad and several invaluable friends. I could never have done it without all of you.

I'm In

Prison

I feel like I am a prisoner,
Watched every minute every day.
I feel trapped and like I'm a burden.
I hate that I feel this way.

I can't even go for a wee in peace,
In case I do sit-ups on the floor.
I'm so cross at this situation,
And ED is so hard to ignore.

My fear of food is debilitating.
I feel like I'm sofa bound.
I've just been given some sausages,
And my heart has started to pound.

I have to psych up myself to eat things,
Like I'm about to jump from a plane.
ED keeps saying don't do it.
This all must sound so insane.

But food is what keeps me going.
It's food that allows me to move.
ED tells me it tastes bad.
I need to shut him away to improve.

This food is actually yummy.
From now on I'll try to ignore.
I'm killing him with every mouthful,
And soon I'll hear him no more.

I know my illness not only made me feel rubbish but that some of the horrible feelings were transferred to those around me too. I know that it must have been a difficult jump for Mike and my mum to become carers for me. My mum came around every weekday to stay with me whilst Mike was at work. This was the only option unless I was to go into an inpatient unit.

Mike would leave for work and I promised myself to stay in bed until my mum arrived at 8.30am. I would dread her knock at the door as that hour felt like the only time I had just for me. Her knock meant starting the day and to me that translated into eating and going through yet another exhausting battle in my head. Mike would care for me in the evenings and at weekends. Saturday was the worst as that was dreaded weigh-in day and this ruled my world for so many months.

About a month into my recovery, my mum started dropping me at Sally's house each week and I'd spend the day with her and her 18-month-old daughter, Jasmine. I really treasured this time, especially as I missed my class of toddlers at school. I'll always look back on the time I spent with them with happy memories and I'm so grateful to Sally for letting me into her world. Seeing Jasmine each week helped to take my mind off ED and focused it on the reasons for recovery. I wanted so desperately to be a mum and I knew that ED wouldn't allow this to happen. I had to choose between ED and being a mum, an easy choice for me to make.

During this period, my parents had to go to India to visit my brother and so Ellie came to stay with me for two weeks to prevent me from having to go into an inpatient unit. Ellie and I have always just got on and she's always understood my quirks. They say every brunette needs a blonde and Ellie is most definitely mine. Unfortunately, about two days into her stay with me, my grandpa was taken ill and we spent every day visiting him for hours in hospital. Ellie sat and held my grandpa's hand and spoke to the doctors with me. My grandpa sadly passed away the day after my parents arrived home. He knew about my anorexia before he died and I hated the thought that he passed away thinking I was poorly. So from that day forward I vowed I would beat ED for him.

Trust has always been of great importance to me. So the thought that I wasn't even trusted to go to the bathroom in case I did a few cheeky sit-ups was so debilitating. My partner, my mum and my friends all had to sit and watch me wee. I can't imagine how strange it must have been for them to see me in this state. Before each meal or snack I would psych myself up as though I was about to do a Bear Grylls challenge. Eventually, I began to enjoy the food I ate. This made ED go crazy! Food gave me energy to think and to do. I could actually watch a forty-minute TV show without thinking about food or exercise. I could sit and read without feeling an ounce of guilt. I was slowly starting to feel more like Georgie again.

What Is

ED?

Most don't seem to understand,
"Well what is ED?"
I guess it's hard to comprehend,
It's not something you can see.

ED's a monster in my head,
With a very wicked voice.
He tells me things and makes me feel,
As though I have no choice.

Every day he chants at me,
"You're worthless! You're no good!
You should eat less. You should run more.
You should, you should, you should!"

If you ask me what he looks like,
You'd think that I were mad.
He's green with sharp points on his back,
Like a Mr Man gone bad.

He has a small, sneaky smile,
And black, beady eyes.
He's a master of disguises,
And a pro at telling lies.

He zaps all of my energy.
Tells me who I need to be.
ED is a killer,
And he's trying to kill me.

I imagine that some of you reading this book may be a bit confused each time I write ED. Some of you will no doubt be thinking, 'who is ED, and why does she refer to him all the time'. Well let me introduce you to ED...

ED is the monster that lives in my head. Call me crazy but he genuinely does. ED is another name for my eating disorder and a way to separate my anorexic thoughts from my own 'normal' thoughts. I don't actually think I am that 'normal' by the way and I think Mike would agree! Everyone is different so 'normal' will look different on each and every one of us. The one thing that I am certain about, however, is that I am definitely far more normal than ED!

ED's favourite things to say include the words fat, worthless and ugly. Sometimes it's like he is stuck on repeat in my head. ED has been around for a lot longer than I first realised. He has been part of my thoughts from quite a young age. He has often made me feel painfully shy and extremely self-conscious, not just about my appearance, but my personality too. I was convinced no one would like me and that I didn't matter to anyone.

I remember telling my psychologist about ED for the first time. I told her that he 'lived' in the left-hand side of my brain - it sounds crazy I know. I had a very clear picture of what ED looked like and still do. He is a little green monster, like a Mr Man crossed with the Grinch. Honestly, he is that horrible! He is spikey and has short little legs that he uses to pace up and down across my mind. I think my mind came up with ED as I have always been a very imaginative person but being able to visualise my eating disorder as a physical thing really helped in my recovery. It meant that I could separate what was ED and what was Georgie.

This ability to separate the two sets of thoughts still helps me to this day. Does Georgie want to go for a walk? Yes? Then go! No? Then stay home. I have learnt to do exactly the opposite of what ED wants. I think that everyone, eating disorder or not, has an unhelpful part to their minds. The part that tells you how you should feel on a day-to-day basis. The difference is that ED was talking over my brain leaving me feeling totally suffocated by him.

We did a lot of work on ED in my sessions, including picturing him as a different colour to make him seem less daunting. Yellow was my chosen colour as it is my favourite and a colour that I associate with feeling happy. I feel that it defines the Georgie I 'lost'. Doing little things like this to change my perception of ED really helped to silence his voice.

We would also challenge ED by using factual information. If ED told me I was useless at life then we would look at the facts. Does having loving family and friends, your ideal job and a roof over your head equate to being useless at life? Facts really helped me to differentiate ED's voice from reality, as all he does is lie.

A Three

Part Key

I have three different professionals,
All three of them are key.
They're helping me get better.
To free me from ED.

My psychiatrist is an older man,
I doubted him at first.
But he's one of the most intelligent men,
And he helped me at my worst.

My dietician is amazing!
She's a scientist at heart.
She knew exactly what I needed,
And has been there from the start.

She put a stop to all my exercise,
And helped me with my diet.
ED did not like this at all,
But it worked, he's now gone quiet.

My psychologist is also fantastic,
She's someone I won't forget.
She's helped me learn to love myself,
And to not live with regret.

I know that I am lucky,
To have access to these three.
If I'd had to wait those three more months,
I don't know where I'd be.

I know how scary it is having professionals 'control' what you do and eat for weeks on end. But I promise you it will turn out to be life changing. I will be forever grateful to the three professionals that took the plunge into recovery with me.

When I first met my psychiatrist, they were definitely not what I had expected but then what do you expect!? I guess it's a bit like expecting every teacher to be like Miss Honey from Matilda but that is near impossible in my opinion. I think I was expecting a young (ish), smart, serious, slightly geeky professional. The reality was an older gentleman who looked as though he had just stepped off a plane from Spain.

To be honest, I initially assumed he was another patient. That was until he cautiously walked towards me, shook my hand and introduced himself. Little did I know back then that he would turn out to be one of the most talented, intelligent, kind men I have ever met. He set me up with both my dietitian and my psychologist. This is something I dreaded at the time — the two people who would basically kill ED. You can imagine what that did to my head!

My dietitian taught me how to fall back in love with nutrition because that's what food is. It helps you to function as a human being. My dietician essentially approached everything from a scientific point of view. I really took note of everything she told me and followed her diet plan to the letter, although this wasn't always easy. I treated her like the goddess of food and would go to her for advice whenever I needed it.

I could never trick her with lies like "I did eat all of that and I haven't done any secret exercise this week". She would always say, "science doesn't lie Georgie, so what have you been doing?" This used to infuriate me but now I look back and smile.

My psychologist was one of the 'rocks' of my recovery. I could never have done it without her support. I dread to think of how many endless moans and stories like 'strawberry day' I have bored her with over the last few years. But I never once felt judged or weird when chatting to her.

I can assure you that some of the things that came out of my anorexia possessed mouth would definitely be classed as weird at the very least! We have spent many sessions laughing and talking through the crazy things that my mind would tell me, making ED feel smaller and smaller as each session went by. By just walking through the door that very first day on the 23rd February 2018, I knew that ED had already started to shrink.

Scales

Scales are the worst thing in the world.
Why do they even exist!?
Why do I care what the number says?
Why do I always resist?

The thing I've come to realise,
Is that scales are just a tool.
And when they ask to weigh me,
They're not trying to be cruel.

It's not a measure of my worth.
It won't define all that I am.
It's not something that I have to pass.
It isn't an exam.

The measure is only useful,
To a medical pro.
No one else, including me,
Really needs to know.

When have I ever opened with,
"Hi, I'm Georgie, I weigh A."
Who would actually care?
Plus it would be really weird to say.

I won't think of my weight at all,
When I'm laid on my death bed.
So, from now on I'm going to live my life,
By experiences instead.

Let's talk about numbers. Numbers ruled my life in every form. Steps, time, volume on the radio, scales, likes, calories, how many mouthfuls of food, how much I spent, everything and anything I would put a number to and be in competition with. It was like I just saw them everywhere and I had to be the best. Ironically, I am now a "maths teacher". I've put it in inverted comma's as anyone who knows me will tell you I'm rubbish at maths but apparently, I can teach it okay to five-year old's, or so I hope!

Numbers are basically a way of keeping control of life but they can easily become an obsession. I have learnt to just let go of keeping track. It started with little things like being one minute late to see a friend. Did they notice? No. Okay, well then it doesn't matter. If they did notice, did anything bad happen? No. Then it doesn't matter. It's the same with everything that you can put a number on. Will doing 1000 more steps make you wake up with the perfect body? No. Well then it doesn't matter! Honestly, it really, really doesn't matter.

I now try and live in the moment. If that means the radio is on an odd number because I want to sing really loudly to a song that's just come on, or if that means having the sandwich I was really craving rather than the one that has a 'good' number on the front, then so be it. Because that is living!

I had, well still sort of have, a difficult relationship with the dreaded scales. I don't like them and probably never will but that doesn't mean I have to live in fear of them. Do I need to know my weight? No. Do I need to be healthy and happy? Yes. I did a lot of work in my sessions about scales. It entailed many rounds of eye movement desensitization and reprocessing (EDMR) therapy. This quite literally opened my eyes to lots of things that I feel I should share:

1. Scales are just a tool that someone created to help medical professionals to better understand our bodies. So that they are able to give us the correct doses of medicine and to measure our health NOT our happiness.

2. Our weight is not our worth.

3. The number isn't important. If it really was that important then we would feel the need to tell everyone. The reality is no one cares. Do you care what your neighbours weigh? I bet you don't. In fact, I bet you have only just thought about it for the first time ever. That's because it doesn't matter!

4. You don't need to know your weight. Do you feel happy and healthy? Are you able to move your body, and partake in experiences? Yes? Then you are living life and that's what's important. No? Then ask for help. Standing on scales alone never helped anyone.

5. When you do happen to see what you weigh don't compare it to anything. Let it go in one ear and out the other then get on with your day.

I've Won

ED is trapped behind thick bars.
I've done it. I have won!
Yes I sometimes hear him,
But now I'm the stronger one.

I feel like now I can live my life.
I'm not trapped anymore.
I've been to amazing places,
And there's still many to explore.

I eat food without thinking of calories.
I wear bikinis and don't give a damn.
My mind's not just focused on exercise,
And I've accepted all that I am.

I can't wait to start a family,
Something I'd never have got with ED.
I'll show my kids a life more than numbers,
And maybe I'll tell them of me.

Being ill and facing up to it,
Was the hardest thing I've done.
I couldn't have come as far as this,
Without support from everyone.

To those who supported me the most,
I'll be forever in your debt.
Now to start my life finally as me,
"Hi, I'm Georgie, we've not met."

I feel so proud of where I have come and I can't wait to share it with you all. I am living proof that you can overcome ED. It's hard, really hard. But you can do it! I can safely say that I now love my life. I am writing this sat on a deckchair in my back garden looking across at a beautiful view. I feel incredibly lucky. Turn back a few years and you would never have seen me sunbathing unless I was on a secluded beach. I have always loved the sun but getting what I previously perceived to be my 'fat tummy' out to the world, only ever happened on rare occasions.

The first holiday I went on after getting help was to Greece with Mike. I remember feeling anxious about every aspect of it. What will I eat? What will I wear? Will I be able to wear my bikini? What will people think of my body? Will I feel anxious the whole week? Will I have to go out for drinks? Some of these may be things that other people worry about before they go away but mine was to the extreme. However, when I got there it felt as though I had left ED in England.

It was one of the first times I felt free. I ate ice cream every day, wore my bikini 95% of the time and went out for countless meals, drinks and pancake's and I absolutely LOVED it. Everyone in Greece in mid-August wears very little. This meant that it left very little to the imagination, which helped me to realise that no one looks the same and no one has these perfect bodies that are printed in magazines. I left Greece with a new sense of normal. Since then, I have really enjoyed going on holiday and my confidence has increased dramatically. I now feel like a new version of 'me'. This Georgie will stand up for herself, not only to ED if he ever tries to creep back up but in work and relationships too.

To a certain degree I am still a 'yes girl'. Saying the word 'no' just doesn't come naturally to me. But I have learnt that sometimes I have to look after myself before I can take care of others. If I strongly disagree with something that someone says to me then I will stand up for myself and voice my opinion. The old Georgie would have just let it fester in her head or worse still, apologised for anything and everything just to prevent an argument.

Now, I literally picture ED behind bars in my head. Yes, I might sound crazy but if there's a chance of helping someone else then I'm fine to admit my quirks! ED does still try and lecture me about steps or calories once in a while but for the most part I can now ignore him and get on with my day. I have learnt that life is for living.

Everyone has bad days and I won't lie to anyone and say that I feel 100% all the time as that would be impossible. Embrace the bad days and use them as an excuse to look after number one. I can't wait to explore more of the world, try new food, get married and start a family all with ED firmly locked behind bars. It's time to say goodbye to ED and hello to Georgie. I'm coming to get you world!

A Message

From Me

To You

The voice in your head is so, so loud.
I feel your pain, I really do.
You live in fear of getting fat,
And ED is taunting you.

If you haven't yet then please, please, please,
Seek help, don't fight alone.
You won't regret it, I promise,
There's so much I wish I'd known.

Fat is something you need to live,
Just like your heart, your lungs, your skin.
Calories feed your body's battery,
And this powers everything.

It's human nature to sometimes be envious,
Of peoples looks and possessions too.
But don't compare yourself to anyone,
As no one else is you!

There can only be one survivor,
In the war of "ED versus me".
The key is to build an army,
To make it "ED versus we".

Now, whenever I feel a little bit down,
There's something I like to sing,
"My name is Georgie Beadman,
And I can do anything!"

I want to finish with some things that I found really helped me during my recovery from ED.

1. Keep your mind constantly busy. Do whatever you can to stop ED sneaking back in. I know this is easier said than done but seriously find a new skill - draw, make jewellery, take up a musical instrument or write a book. This is exactly what I did. With the help of Sally, I co-wrote my first children's book 'The Potogold and the Broken Rainbow'. I then went on to publish a second children's book by myself 'DooDoo the Doodlebug'. This is another reason I have to be thankful for Sally. She gave me the writing buzz. For a girl who is heavily dyslexic and struggled at school this was quite the achievement and something I am immensely proud of. So, if there's something you want to try then give it a go and don't let anyone tell you that you can't!

2. Don't listen to anyone else's opinion on food other than your dietitian or psychologist. I often found facts about food confusing and didn't know who to trust. ED would convince me that some people were telling me what I wanted to hear rather than the truth. I remember my dietitian telling me once that she was a scientist and had studied food for years. She made me promise not to take advice from anyone except her about my food intake. I have now downloaded this to my brain and only take food advice from myself and myself only. ED stays well behind his bars and I ignore anything he tries to tempt me with. If I fancy chocolate, I have chocolate. If I fancy an apple, I have an apple.

3. Be yourself! All human beings are different and we are all amazing. If people don't like you for you then that's fine. Go and make friends with someone else who does. Not all puzzle pieces fit together.

4. Try to see yourself as others see you and accept any compliments that people give you. Write them down in a book and look at them on a rainy day.

5. Surround yourself with positive people. Don't be afraid to admit that you are struggling. That's what friends and family are for. Never suffer alone.

6. Don't let ED fool you into lying about anything. Tell the people you trust the most the honest truth so that they can support you. ED feeds off lies so make sure you starve him and not yourself.

7. Don't feel guilty for anything. Guilt was a huge part of my illness. If you have sat on the sofa all day, not spoken to anyone and then eaten a takeaway that's okay! Your body was probably in need of a rest and time to refuel. You should not feel any guilt for feeding your body and taking time out for you.

8. Live life and keep smiling. I'll finish with a quote from Dory – 'just keep swimming' and all will be okay. I promise.

She Can
She Will
She Did

The Girl With

The Alphabet

Leggings

She's wearing alphabet leggings.
Her hair is effortlessly done.
She's such a bubbly person.
She seems like so much fun.

Perhaps she is a foreigner,
That might explain her style.
"Hi", I introduce myself.
She replies with a smile.

She's just asked if I will join her,
At the food fest in the street.
"We could go and have a wander,
Perhaps have a bite to eat."

We head down to the stalls,
And find lots of types of cheese.
"I can't I'm lactose intolerant,
But you go ahead, please."

Oo yum a brownie stand.
"Ahh they're not gluten free."
There's lots of gin to sample.
"No thanks, that's not for me."

"Poor girl", I think to myself,
As we continue through the crowd.
She has so many allergies,
There's so much she's not allowed.

ELLIE

Georgie, Georgina, G, Doo-Doo - all names that I've known my amazing friend by. But, back in the beginning, she was 'The Girl with the Alphabet Leggings'. And we still refer to that name fondly even now. I met Georgie on day two of starting out on our own big adventures. We were both studying Primary Teaching at York St. John University and we were equally excited, nervous and desperate to make friends. Well that day, I made one of my lifelong friends who, further down the line, I would hold hands with on an incredible, often painful and ultimately life-changing journey.

We had just been put into our classes and were being given a tour of the place we were set to call home for the next three years. As I wandered shyly around the grounds with the other twenty students in my group, I noticed what could only be described as a ray of sunshine up ahead. A girl wearing alphabet leggings, clearly as clueless as I was as to who anyone was. Her hair was effortlessly done in that 'bed head but looks great' way and her skin was so olive that I was convinced she was Italian. "Hi", I said. "Hi, I'm Georgie", she beamed back at me. She was not Italian, she was very, very British!

Reflecting back on this with all that has happened in the last seven years, I am so happy that Georgie can now see herself in the way I saw her that day. A beautiful, vivacious character with a zest for life so strong it burned out of her and a sense of individual style that made her stand out from the crowd in all the right ways. We stuck together that day. We sat together in class, found our way around university and when we finished early from lectures Georgie suggested we could go to the food festival in town and get some late lunch. Oh how ironic it is that this is where our journey started.

Both new to the City of York, we found our way into the centre and immersed ourselves amongst the chaos and aromas of the annual food festival in the square. We had a look at the chutneys and I sampled the cheese. "I can't have cheese as I'm lactose intolerant but you go ahead," she told me. We found the brownie stand - "Ahh none of them are gluten free but you have one, they look amazing", she remarked. We found the local gin stall - "I'm not a fan of gin but you go ahead, that raspberry one looks good!" We stumbled across the stone baked pizza samples - "There's gluten AND dairy in that so I'll have to miss out but try that pepperoni one if you want, it looks good."

I remember thinking, "oh the poor girl, she has so many allergies." We finally settled on buying lunch from the hog roast stall. A floury bap for me crammed full with juicy pork, crackling, stuffing and lashings of apple sauce. Then a tray full of the meat and sauce for my new companion. And there it started. The trips to town, the lunches out, the evening meals, all with the new best friend who couldn't eat cheese, wouldn't try brownies and refused a shot of alcohol that was being given away for free.

It's Just

Georgie

It's strange how when I met her,
I felt an instant click.
She's just one of those people,
You warm to really quick.

Dinners out and cocktail nights,
Have become our new routine.
All organised by Georgie,
She's such the social Queen.

She always orders salads,
And she'll never choose a main.
I assume it's as her allergies,
Would cause her stomach pain.

She won't drink any alcohol.
She says she doesn't like the taste.
So the 2 for 1 cocktail nights,
Seem like such a waste.

She's also quite a fidget.
She's always on the go.
Why she can't just sit for lunch,
I really do not know.

All this is just who Georgie is.
She's different, like her style.
But she's become one of my closest friends,
And she always makes me smile.

ELLIE

We were best friends from that first day and, along with Georgie's new flat mate, Amy, as well as a few of the girls from lectures, our social life was formed. That social life often consisted of lunches and early bird dinners at our favourite restaurants or 2 for 1 cocktails. It might seem strange to hear that this was how we socialised considering you're reading a book about overcoming an eating disorder but food and drink were always a big part of our friendship. Georgie was just VERY good at hiding things at the time.

We all knew Georgie was dairy and lactose intolerant so no one batted an eyelid when the waiter would come over and she would say, "I'll just have the starter sized Caeser salad but with no cheese or croutons and can you bring it out with the mains please." Why did we never question that she always went for a starter size? I don't know. It was just normal for her. Georgie couldn't eat bread, she couldn't drink milk and she didn't like alcohol.

Yes of course I notice the patterns now. The patterns slap me in the face but back then, they didn't. She seemed to genuinely enjoy going out for lunch. She would be the ringleader in organising the 2 for 1 cocktail nights and it was more often than not Georgie who suggested movie nights with strawberries, chocolates and marshmallows. So, between her sunny demeanor, zest for life and apparent love of food, an eating disorder never even entered our heads. Or if it did, it was soon pushed away with the thought, "No not Georgie. That happens to other people not my best friend." Looking back though, it wasn't just food. It was patterns and behaviours. When the other girls in our friendship group would head to the common room, the canteen or SU bar to tuck into their sandwiches at lunch, Georgie and I would head into town. Not to visit a pub or a restaurant but to..... well, honestly, I don't know what to do. It was all so that she could spend our hours lunch break on the go. Constantly moving, walking into town, nipping around the shops. It was always done under the pretense of, "Ellie you haven't brought lunch today have you? Shall we go to the shop in town so you can buy your favourite salmon sandwich."

We would often go and visit the Nut Shop. An Aladdin's cave tucked away down a cobbled street with jars full of chocolate covered peanuts, banana chips, yoghurt raisins and more. I was always partial to a big bag of Bombay mix or chocolate covered ginger and Georgie loved a pick'n'mix bag of dried fruit, seeds and nuts. The difference between us though was that mine was devoured with a can of coke or a coffee as an afternoon snack, hours after I'd enjoyed a proper lunch, whereas Georgie's bag of fruit and nuts was her lunch. That was it. And that bag would last her days. A small portion rationed off each day for lunch. And she could only allow herself to have that ration if she'd run a distance that she felt was deserving of lunch.

Always

Running

Wow she runs a lot.
She must be very fit!
I've never been a runner,
I much prefer to sit.

She must be training for a marathon,
With the miles she runs each day.
It seems a bit excessive,
But then, who am I to say?

In winter she'll be up and out,
Way before the sun.
I know I'm not a runner,
But that doesn't seem like fun.

I've noticed she's quite grumpy,
If she hasn't clocked her miles.
But as soon as she's had her fix,
She's back to being all smiles.

It seems like an addiction.
She's always on the go.
But again, I'm not a runner,
So I suppose how would I know?

ELLIE

If someone had asked me to summarise Georgie it would be, "Well she's very close to her family, she loves working with children, her main hobby is running (she's really fit), she likes handbags and loves pick'n'mix sweets." So, you see, running was just Georgie. Yes, she ran every day but to be honest, I wasn't a runner so I didn't know that wasn't normal.

What we didn't know at the time was that, for Georgie, running meant she was allowed to eat that day. I don't know how her mindset worked exactly but from what she has told me since it was — as long as the run was the right length then she could allow herself lunch and dinner that day. If she had something coming up like a meal out or girly cocktail evening then the run had to be extra-long. If something prevented her from running for as long one day then she could only have fruit for breakfast, certainly no yoghurt, and lunch would have to be skipped too. She once told me that she would feel angry all day if she hadn't run. Was that an alarm bell? No not at the time. To me it was - Georgie runs, she loves it and that was all there was to it. Should it have been? Yes, it definitely should!

During our final year at university Georgie met Mike. It's funny when your bestie gets a new boyfriend isn't it. You feel like you know the poor guy inside out before he and your friend have even been on their first date! Mike was the older guy that we pawed over on Tinder who I helped her compose messages to. After university all the

76

girls moved back home with their parents whilst they saved for houses or for travelling. Georgie was the first to jump the initial hurdle in the big game of adult life. Yep, she was the first one of all the girls to buy a house and she was buying it with Mike. Wow life was really looking good for G! But it didn't stay like that for long and running was the cause.

I distinctly remember the first conversation I had with Georgie where I really didn't understand her running obsession. She was telling me how her and Mike couldn't see eye to eye about the fact that she had to stop on the way home for a run. "Sorry if I'm ranting," she seethed at me down the phone, "but he just doesn't get it! You get it don't you? I have to stop and run for an hour on the way home because I don't get time in the morning and well....if I didn't do it then when would I?! And yes, it means I get home much later in the evenings and Mike and I don't get as much time together and dinner is much later than it needs to be but, Ellie, you can see I've got no choice. I have to run for an hour on the way home. I have to!"

But why did she? Couldn't she just run at the weekends and stop what was obviously becoming an obsession and eating away at her relationship? When I think back to that conversation, I think that was the point where it started to subconsciously click with both of us that something wasn't right here. Should I have been concerned at that point and intervened? Yes! Yes of course! But at the time that was Georgie. Just Georgie.

She Has An

Eating

Disorder

I've just been told the news,
And I'm actually quite in shock.
Georgie? No not Georgie!
She's always been a rock.

She's been battling on for years,
But no else has known.
Then yesterday she blurted out,
"I can't do this alone."

She has an eating disorder,
And she's really very sick.
She's waiting now to get some help.
I hope she gets it quick.

I can't imagine what she's been through.
It must have been so hard.
It must have taken so much effort,
To keep holding up her guard.

It really makes me sad that she,
Has fought this for so long.
I feel ashamed I didn't notice,
That things were very wrong.

I wish she'd told me sooner,
Not tried so hard to hide.
But at least she's asked for help now,
And I'll be right by her side.

ELLIE

"Hmmm I think Georgie might be pregnant." I speculated excitedly to my partner Tom. Of course, he dismissed it and said he hadn't noticed anything, but something wasn't quite right about her behaviour and what she had told me on the phone.

It was our first year spending New Year's Eve together. Georgie and Mike had travelled to my parents' house where we had spent a games night with my parents and siblings. She hadn't had a drink all night (which wasn't unusual for G) and as usual we had catered to her 'dietary requirements' of dairy and gluten free, but for anything that she hadn't been able to eat she politely said how it didn't matter and she'd be fine.

It was the conversation I had with her the next day on the phone that really did it. "I've realised something about myself. I am going to tell you but we want to tell our parents first." I thought the deal was sealed; she was definitely having a baby. How exciting!

Never. Never in a million years did I expect what it really was. Never did I expect to be told that actually she was unwell. Never did I think I'd hear her say, "It's like a lightbulb has gone off in my head. I have an unhealthy relationship with food and I'm obsessed with running."

I was devasted. Devastated for her that her whole world was about to flip. Devastated that as her friend I hadn't realised. And devastated that the news I thought was about to be so lovely, so beautifully life changing, was in fact the exact opposite.

She was still her though. She was still Georgie Beadman. Still Doo-Doo. She hadn't had a personality transplant. She was still Georgie who loved her yellow hoodie she bought in Devon, who wore a multitude of rings and laughed at how blunt and honest she could be. My best friend didn't change when she admitted this.

If you're reading this from my perspective, as a friend or family member of someone with an eating disorder, they won't change either. Your friend, your sister, your brother, your child - they are still there. You can still laugh about the same things. They just need your understanding and support.

Georgie and I laughed about how her timing couldn't have been worse as I was about to go travelling six weeks after she told me so I wouldn't be there for a big chunk of her recovery. And so, we made the decision that her and her mum, Fiona, would come and stay with me in a local B&B for two nights. That way we could see each other before I went away.

How Did I

Not Know?

I still can't quite believe it.
I just don't understand.
Why did I not notice,
Before it got so out of hand?

There were so many little clues,
Now that I think back.
She'd rarely ever eat her lunch,
And she'd never have a snack.

She used all of her "allergies",
To justify what she ate.
But she'd always been so skinny,
I didn't register her weight.

I suppose all of her running,
Should have set off an alarm.
But I just thought she enjoyed it,
I didn't see the harm.

She seemed to have such zest for life,
She always wore a grin.
I'd never have imagined,
Her battles from within.

I feel guilty that I didn't clock,
Many years ago.
How did I not see it?
How did I not know?

SALLY

On the handful of times that I'd met Georgie prior to her diagnosis I had noticed she had her quirks. It didn't matter whether it was snowing, raining or scorching hot she would always be wearing a baggy coat, usually teamed with a loose pair of shorts. I could tell that she was very much an outdoor type so I just put her choice of style down to this. She seemed like the kind of person who would do well on a Bear Grylls show - I actually found out from Georgie at a later date that she had in fact applied for one of his shows!

I think it was the second time I met her that we all went for coffee and cake after a walk. It was then that she told us she couldn't eat cake because she was allergic to gluten. I told her that they also served some really good ice creams and she replied that she couldn't have those either as she was lactose intolerant. Ashamedly, I will admit that I did an inward eye roll at this point. I thought to myself, "Oh no Mike has found himself another high maintenance one who likes fad diets." I look back and want to slap myself for thinking like that.

When I first found out that Georgie had an eating disorder all these little quirks I'd noticed began to make sense. I would never have added them up to an eating disorder but I told myself it was because I didn't know her well enough. However, something that I failed to understand at the time, which is probably something most people will also wonder, was how did those who were closer to her not notice? How did they not know?

Yes, how did I not know? I ask myself that question a lot. But honestly, it was not obvious. The biggest thing I have learnt since Georgie has been in recovery is that people with an eating disorder are Olympic gold medalists in the art of deception. Second only to their skill of getting through the day on a dangerously low number of calories. You see to me, people with an eating disorder had some very clear red flags and Georgie had none.

People with an eating disorder avoided food at all costs and would never suggest meals out, girly cocktail nights or movie nights with hot chocolate and snacks. They wouldn't say the best thing about a trip to the cinema was getting there early to peruse the pick'n'mix selection and cram as much as they could into the overpriced paper bags.

What's more, people with severe mental health problems are not the life and soul of the party. They aren't the ray of sunshine that Georgie was. They didn't go out of the way to help others, have a zest for life that meant our weekends were full of day trips and nights out all organised by her. That was the Georgie that I and all those that loved her knew. How wrong we were!

It wasn't until four years later that I discovered that yes, Georgie had been and done all of those things. She was wonderful. But she was also poorly, really poorly, and struggling. She was the queen of hiding the truth. And I didn't know. I never knew. How did I not know?

I Just Don't Understand

"An evil, invisible monster",
That's how she describes ED.
But accepting this explanation,
Is proving difficult for me.

I am trying really, really hard,
Not to lose my shit.
But it feels like everything I say,
Is drowned out by this twit.

"Why don't we watch a movie?
A chick flick might be fun."
But she is looking out the window,
Clearly thinking she should run.

I put her plate down on the table,
A simple lunch of beans on toast.
And honestly, you would probably think,
That she'd just seen a ghost.

I'm trying hard to be patient,
And to hold my anger in.
But sometimes I do wonder,
Does she even want to win?

I wish I could come face to face,
With this monster called ED.
I'd kick and scream and shout "fuck off",
Leave my Georgie be!

SALLY

Supporting someone with an eating disorder takes A LOT of patience. I can't say it takes understanding because, unless you've had an eating disorder, it's not something you can understand. Georgie found a warped sense of comfort in hunger. I hate being hungry. It makes me feel shakey and faint so I just didn't get it!

The only way for Georgie to improve her physical health was for her to increase her food intake. Georgie knew this and yet she still resisted. She would sit for what felt like hours psyching herself up to eat a sandwich and a packet of crisps for lunch. It took all the patience I had (and this is a lot bearing in mind I had an 18-month-old) not to shake her and say, "it's only a packet of crisps!"

At various stages in her recovery Georgie was set challenges by her dietician. One of these was to try and enjoy a cake and a chat with me. This was a normal weekly activity for me but for Georgie, it was a big event. I sat and scoffed mine without even thinking about it. Meanwhile, Georgie proceeded to tell me the longest story ever. I can't even remember what the story was about, I just remember thinking that it was a blatant stall technique. I began to feel extremely uncomfortable as the longer her story went on the more this cupcake in front of her became a huge elephant in the room. In the end she ate it. I don't know whether she enjoyed the cake or not but it left me feeling extremely tense. It was only then that I began to realise what it must be like for her.

ELLIE

Georgie was coming to visit me with her mum before I went away for four months. That was the first blow. She wasn't hopping on a train or driving her yellow KA and coming for a girl's weekend with her bestie. She was coming with her mum to be looked after 24/7. The second blow came when I saw her. It had only been about four weeks since she'd told me but, in that time, she'd completely succumbed to ED's voice. I wasn't prepared for how much weight she'd lost. It was so obvious even through all the layers she was wearing.

I knew she was surviving on practically nothing but seeing it with my own eyes was painful. That was blow number three. I watched my best friend sustain herself on a pint of Diet Coke after going for a two-hour run. In the evenings, whilst we were ordering delicious three course meals, Georgie was tucking into her first edible substance of the day - vegetables, with added emphasis for no sauces, no dressings and absolutely no butter. It was heart-breaking. It was shocking.

You might read this and wonder why we let it happen. Why we allowed her, as her mum and her best friend, to go all day on only Diet Coke and let her run for miles. Our job, as the people who loved her, was to support her and make sure she trusted us. Would she have still trusted us and been open and honest if we had looked at her choices disapprovingly? Of course not. Help was coming. Our role was to love her and be there until that help began.

How Do

I Help?

Saying, "I need help",
Was hard for her to do.
But how exactly I can help her,
I haven't got a clue.

I could shower her with compliments.
Remind her that she's tough.
But she probably wouldn't have it,
And it doesn't seem enough.

I cannot make her better,
By forcing her to eat.
And she wouldn't take it kindly,
If I tied her to her seat.

I could send her thoughtful gifts,
That say, "I'm thinking of you!"
But really, what good are these,
With what she's going through.

She needs to build her strength up,
To win the battle with ED.
She needs to know she's not alone.
She has a team now. She has me.

So, instead I'll simply hold her hand,
And offer her my ear.
I'll give her all the time I have,
And let her know I'm here.

ELLIE

I was in contact with Georgie most days during my travels. We chatted about where I'd been and what I was seeing and what she'd been up to with her mum. We also chatted about ED. She would tell me how hard it was, what it felt like and what thoughts she had. About half way through my travels Georgie's mum, Fiona, messaged to say she was going to visit Georgie's brother for two weeks and wondered if I could stay with Georgie when I was back. It was sad to think that the reason for me staying the fortnight was because she was too sick to be on her own.

I'd been home for about three weeks when I headed to Georgie's. There was no denying the fact that she was ill but those two weeks were not about her condition. They were not about being a carer. They were about having fun again and enjoying each other's company. I really don't look back on those two weeks and think of ED. Yet he was there and G was still very much in the thick of her battle with him.

There were quite a few rules regarding food. She wasn't allowed to make it herself, there were certain things that had to be eaten at breakfast, lunch and dinner. Snacks were also part of the routine. It was so wonderful to see her eating naturally though. Her new routine was exactly what I did anyway so, to me, it just felt like a lovely time with my best friend. Despite all the loveliness and fun we had though, I knew that a big responsibility rested on my shoulders that fortnight.

SALLY

My biggest frustration was wanting to help but not knowing how. If Georgie had broken her leg, I could have helped by carrying things for her. If she had been diagnosed with cancer, I could have gone along to chemotherapy sessions and held her hand. However, Georgie's battle was with her own head. It wasn't something you could see or even visualise. It wouldn't have shown up on a medical scan and it wasn't something that was easy to explain. The only way in which to quantify or measure the effect that it was having on her was to weigh her and this act in itself sent Georgie spiraling back down.

She had been fighting this battle alone for such a long time that I'm not sure Georgie even knew what we could do to help. Given how well she had hidden things, it was also hard to know whether she was actually doing okay or whether it was another front.

Eventually, I came to realise that the best way to help Georgie was to try and act as normal as possible around her. For a long time, she couldn't be left on her own but that didn't mean we couldn't do normal things together during that time. In fact, we actually got really into creative activities and in the weeks leading up to Christmas we must have made nearly a hundred Brussel sprout pompoms, which we sold at a craft fair for charity. It sounds like a really random thing to do but it gave Georgie something to focus on. Something positive!

Will I Always Be Suspicious?

I know absolutely none of this,
Was ever Georgie's fault,
But if I say that I don't trust her,
I'd be rubbing her wound with salt.

She became so good at hiding the truth,
She could have won a prize.
But now I find it hard to know,
If she's feeding me more lies.

I don't mean to sound so nasty,
I just worry for my friend.
Will she truly beat ED?
Will this ever end?

I feel tense whilst she places her order,
Whenever we go out for food,
And I struggle not to think the worst,
Whenever she's in a bad mood.

I'm hoping all this will just take time,
That my worries will soon slip away.
In the meantime, I'll just keep quiet.
I wouldn't even know what to say.

SALLY

Trust is something that Georgie really values, as I suppose most people do. But it was really hard to trust her 100%. I hadn't really known Georgie before her diagnosis. All I knew was that she'd been a pro at covering things up. During the months that Georgie wasn't allowed to be left alone it was easy to take her word on things as there was always a witness. It was when she started to gain some freedom again that I began to over-analyse everything she told me.

I once met Georgie early afternoon at a soft play. I'd had lunch before we left the house but during the course of the afternoon it came out in conversation that Georgie had been shopping before coming to meet us. And just like that all I could think was, "she's skipped lunch". I didn't say anything, perhaps I should have, but I felt awful that I didn't trust her. So, I chose to stay quiet.

Another time we stopped for lunch during a walk. I ordered food for myself and my daughter but Georgie just ordered a drink. I started to panic wondering how to handle the situation. Then my little girl said, "Georgie, why aren't you eating?" Oh to have the candor of a small child! She replied that she just hadn't chosen from the menu yet and then went to order something. I was so relieved that the situation had resolved itself but it left me wondering whether I would always be so suspicious. On reflection now, I should have just asked her. I should have been honest. Afterall, honesty is what I was expecting from her.

One particular time that springs to mind is when we were visiting her Grandpa in hospital. We visited him most days during my stay and he was up on a high floor of the hospital. Georgie automatically chose to scale four flights of stairs on the first day we went to visit.

On the following visit, as she headed towards the stairs again, I suggested to her that perhaps we should take the lift. That perhaps, during her recovery, she shouldn't be opting to scale four flights of stairs every day. And do you know what, she agreed with me. She then fell about laughing at how I had totally seen straight through her sneakiness. One thing that G and I often say is that if you don't laugh, you'll cry, and that was something we were not afraid to do.

Since revealing her long-kept secret about ED I'm lucky that Georgie has been very open and honest with me. It's one of the things on a long, long list of things that I'm proud of her for. Throughout her recovery she never hid anything from me, never pretended. She was real and raw and honest. I've really appreciated this as it helped me to better understand what she was going through.

Her honesty about her thoughts and feelings also helped me to be blunt and honest with her. I was able to call her out if ever I thought she was trying to be sneaky. And I can't tell you how much laughter makes a difference in any situation!

She Is

Doing It

Her diagnosis was a shock.
How did I not see?
Yet somehow, this next phase,
Has still crept up on me.

The realisation has now hit,
With something I just saw.
She has put ED in a jail cell,
All that's left is to close the door.

I've had to give myself a pinch,
To check that I'm awake.
She's done it without prompting.
Georgie is eating a cake!

She's now talking of her future,
Of the things she wants to see.
She's excited that perhaps one day,
She'll be a mum like me.

I'm feeling quite emotional.
My eyes are filling with tears.
Finally, she is winning,
After fighting alone for years.

SALLY

Georgie was diagnosed with an eating disorder in January and it was around March time that she started spending one or two days a week with myself and my little girl. Her recovery was a slow and steady process so I never really saw any dramatic changes week to week.

I guess if I had stopped and reflected back at any point then I would have seen a massive improvement but when you're in the midst of it you don't really see the changes. I suppose it's similar to seeing a child grow and develop. The parents don't notice the changes as much compared to someone who only sees them occasionally.

About six months into Georgie's recovery we arranged a weekend away to Windsor with Mike, my husband and my little girl. It was during this trip that I realised just how far Georgie had come. We went to a coffee shop and she ordered and ate a cream cake without any prompting. We had pasta for dinner (her biggest food fear) and she finished the plate. She took my little girl off to the ice cream van and they returned with one each, both beaming with excitement.

I'm not saying this was the end of her recovery process, far from it, but this was the first time that I stood back and thought, "YES GIRL, you're doing it!" Her hair had got it's bounce back, the colour had returned to her cheeks and she looked far less gaunt. She was winning and I couldn't be more proud of her!

Waving goodbye to Georgie to go travelling was the hardest goodbye I've ever experienced. I was about to jet off to the other side of the world for four months for the trip of a lifetime. All the while leaving one of my favourite people behind ready to fight for her life.

When I said "see you soon" to the girl I knew so well, yet also barely recognised, I was so worried that she wouldn't be there when I got back. Whether that was physically or metaphorically, I was terrified that the Georgie I knew would be gone. All I could think was, "Please fight G. Please be here with your sunshiney smile when I get back."

I was so honoured to be asked to stay with Georgie for those two weeks. To be with her, support her and cook for her. Yet, I wasn't caring for her. It didn't feel like that at all because during that fortnight she showed herself to be independent. She was a force to be reckoned with. She was fighting ED with all she had. She was brave, determined and dignified. Even in her weaker moments, to me, she was so strong.

The Georgie I knew and loved was still there. She was well on her way to ridding herself of ED for good. She was winning!

So

Proud

Dare I even say this,
But I think that she has won.
Of course, ED's still in there,
But now she's the stronger one.

Now, there's nothing to stop her.
Her life is back on track.
She's free to do as she wants,
Without the weight of ED on her back.

She used to have to psych herself up,
To eat things plain and small.
Now, she's open to all new foods.
She'll happily try them all.

She can now enjoy some exercise,
Without it controlling her day.
Like a leisurely walk in the country,
With pub lunch along the way.

She has beaten the evil monster,
That no one else could see.
She has won the war she titled,
"ED versus me".

To my beautiful, strong, courageous friend,
I'll forever be in awe.
I have never been so proud of you,
And I couldn't love you more.

ELLIE

The biggest thing I want to emphasise about this journey is that you as the friend, parent or care giver, as well as your loved one battling with mental illness, you don't have to change. Underneath it all, they're still them. It's your job to show them that you are the friend they need, not ED. ED was never their friend. They might have thought he was, but he wasn't. He was just very cunning and sly. Just be there waiting for them when they kick ED out for good. Show them how proud you are. And G how I am proud of you!

That girl in the alphabet leggings is still there. She's always been there. But I can share a pizza with that girl now! I can buy us both an ice cream when we're out on a hot day and make her my favourite pasta dish. She still isn't keen on alcohol unless it's laced with sugar, flavoured with bubble gum and topped with a gummy bear but I know that's just her childish palette that will probably never change and we love her for it! She enjoys Zumba now, not for the calories but for the fun and the laughter. She knows how glorious a Sunday morning lie-in can be followed by a lazy day watching films. Her confidence beams out of her and she truly knows her worth.

Above all else, I hope that she will forever more look in the mirror and see that beautiful ray of sunshine shining back at her. The one I see whenever I look at her, and the one I saw for the first time, when I met the girl in the alphabet leggings.

SALLY

It would be so easy to refer to her now as "the new Georgie". There is so much about her that seems to have changed but the truth is, this Georgie has been there all along. It's just that previously she was suppressed by ED. She is the same bubbly, loving person she always was. But she has far more self-worth now and that in turn feeds her confidence levels and her desire to stand up for herself more. She no longer goes along with what everyone else says. Before, it was as though she was incapable of making decisions. She would always agree with everyone just to keep the peace, probably because she was locked in a constant argument in her head.

I don't think any words can describe how proud we all are of what she's achieved. Personally, I am in total awe of her. She's up there with people who climb Mount Everest in my mind. She's proven herself to have the strength and determination to face anything! She is an amazing role model and has been, and continues to be, a huge positive influence in both my little girls' lives.

In a way I'm thankful to ED as he's the one who brought Georgie and I together. We've been through so much and she's now one of my closest friends and trusted confidants. I can't wait to see what adventures are in store for Georgie. Hopefully one of these will be the great parenting adventure as she will be a brilliant mummy. The main thing is that she is free and the world is now hers for the taking!

You Can And You Will

We all just wanted to leave a final message to anyone who might be reading this book. If you are suffering in a battle with ED at the moment, you've got this! Seriously, you have! ED is a nobody. He doesn't rule over you, you rule over him. Go show everyone what you are made of. Believe Georgie when she says that if you're strong enough to exercise endlessly, starve your body and refuse all of life's little pleasures then you are more than strong enough to stand up to ED.

If someone you love is fighting a battle with ED, then you've got this too! It's not easy looking after someone who has so little self-worth and listens to the monster in their head 90% of the time. But you are more than well equipped to help them. Don't be scared, don't worry that you might say or do the wrong thing. Be honest with how you're feeling too and ask questions. If you open up to them then in all likelihood, they will do the same to you. We asked Georgie so many questions and she was always happy to answer.

Be patient and try to stay calm. We know how hard that can be as it is such a frustrating situation. But confrontation only serves to feed ED. Georgie openly admits that if anyone confronted her or asked her about things directly, she would strongly deny anything was wrong and try to push them away.

Just let them know that you care and will stand by them no matter what. Be accepting - accept their emotions and don't judge them for their actions. Empathy shouldn't be confused with sympathy. It's not about feeling sorry for them, it's about empathising with their emotions and sitting in the moment with them. Let them know that their feelings are valid. Be yourself and take them back to the reasons why you love them. Laugh a lot, let them cry, listen when they explain and cheer when they succeed.

Model natural, normal eating and try to avoid conversations focused around food and exercise. Instead focus on life in general. Try to get them to ask for help on their own terms. This often helps in recovery as their head has started to see the light and is prepared for change. If you get really concerned contact your GP and/or mental health organisation or phone 111/999 in an emergency.

Finally, remember to take time for you! Don't let ED consume all of your energy too. Self-care is important for everyone in this situation not just the sufferer. You are doing an amazing job!!

To those who want to help in other ways...just be a positive role model in society. Don't share fad diets and manic exercise regimes. Be healthy and happy in your own skin. Show people that we all have body hang ups. Embrace your imperfections. They are what make you YOU! Teach children the importance of self-worth and body positivity. Most of all, don't judge. You never know what someone is going through. Let's teach everyone to be themselves and hopefully the world will catch up!

Printed in Great Britain
by Amazon